Table of Contents

Introduction

The Pritikin diet is a low-calorie, low-protein, high-carbohydrate eating plan that recommends a fat intake as low as 10 percent of your daily calories. Developed in the 1970s by Nathan Pritikin, the program is designed to help lower your risk of heart disease, and many of its guidelines have been advocated by the American Heart Association. Although Diet.com reports that the Pritikin diet is linked to lower blood cholesterol, lower blood pressure and a decrease in your chance of obesity, diabetes and certain cancers, its restrictions on what you're allowed to eat may be difficult for some dieters to follow for long periods of time. Talk to your doctor before beginning the Pritikin diet.

The late nutritionist Nathan Pritikin first introduced his low-fat Pritikin Program for Diet and Exercise in 1979, a plan he originally developed for himself to combat heart disease.Robert Pritikin continues his father's work through his own books including ,The New Pritikin Program and The Pritikin Weight Loss Breakthrough.

How the pritikin principle works

The Pritikin Principle is a super-low-fat diet

In a traditionally healthy diet, fat makes up 20 to 30 percent of what you eat. The Pritikin weight-loss program keeps fat under 10 percent. The idea behind this diet is that if you stick to it, you can eat as much as you want and still lose weight.

In addition to being very low in fat, the Pritikin Principle is very high in carbohydrates. You are encouraged to eat lots of fruits, vegetables, and high-fiber grains frequently during the day, an approach that lets you lose weight because you're lowering your calorie intake and reducing your appetite with filling foods. The Pritikin Principle also encourages stress reduction, exercise, and strong social support.

Medical use of the pritikin diet

The Pritikin diet was first designed for prevention and treatment of cardiovascular disease by lowering cholesterol and blood pressure. It has also been promoted as a weight-loss diet and to control blood glucose in patients with prediabetes and type 2 diabetes. Adhering to a low-fat diet leads to overall calorie reduction unless high-fat foods are supplemented with refined carbohydrates and sugar. If vegetables and legumes are eaten instead of refined carbohydrates, then low-fat calorie reduction occurs. The difficulty of this approach is that long-term adherence requires a willingness to avoid many foods and adhere to a strict regimen.

Does the pritikin diet improve health?

The Pritikin diet results in reduction in cholesterol by reducing not only cholesterol intake but also overall caloric intake by limiting all high-fat, calorie-dense foods. Currently, long-term data of the effect of the Pritikin diet on mortality, cardiovascular disease, cancer, and other chronic disease risks are lacking.

Individuals who wish to prevent and treat cardiovascular disease with a very structured and rigid approach may benefit from the Pritikin diet. For patients with prediabetes or type 2 diabetes, the limitation of fat and cholesterol may not be enough to control blood glucose. It is important to consume complex carbohydrates from whole grains, vegetables, and fruits and limit starches.

Potential risks and side effects

The Pritikin diet was designed in the 1970s based on the belief that fat is unhealthy and is the major risk factor for overall health and heart disease. More recently, the adverse effect of added sugars in the diet has become evident. In the first 2 weeks of the diet, significant increases in urine production and fluid shifts may require adjustment of medications for hypertension, heart failure, and diabetes. It is important to consult with a physician before trying the Pritikin diet and to change your diet under the supervision of a physician and a registered dietitian.

The pritikin principle: sample menu

This weight-loss program gets most of its calories from carbohydrates and restricts processed foods, fats, caffeine, sweets, and alcohol. This sample menu contains about 1,200 calories, which break down to 20 percent protein, 70 percent carbohydrates, and less than 10 percent fat:

Breakfast: one-half cup of oatmeal with some jam, one cup of nonfat yogurt, one cup of nonfat milk, and one cup of caffeine-free chicory coffee

• Morning snack: one-half of a whole-wheat bagel and one-half of a cantaloupe

• Lunch: one baked potato with one-half cup of marinara sauce, mixed greens salad, fresh fruit, and a whole-wheat roll

• Afternoon snack: one-half cup of raw broccoli, one-half cup of cauliflower, and two tablespoons of ranch dressing

• Dinner: chicken curry, one cup of asparagus, mixed salad greens, one-half cup of wild rice, one-half cup of skim milk, and one tablespoon of chutney

The pritikin principle: pros and cons

Because the media have largely focused on the low-fat aspects of his diet, most people don't realize that Pritikin also said no to sugar, white flour, and all processed foods, and yes to fresh raw foods, whole grains, and vigorous exercise, A diet low in fat may also protect you from heart disease and some types of cancer. you can lose one to two pounds per week if you exercise and follow his diet.

Disadvantages to the Pritikin Principle are that it is very regimented and may be hard to follow. Also the absence of fat can lead to not getting enough essential fatty acids.

Other possible disadvantages include:

• This plan may be short on vitamins D, E, and B12.

• High-fiber foods can cause digestive disturbance in some people.

• The absence of sugar, salt, and fat can make this diet too bland for some people.

• This diet may lower your good cholesterol.

The pritikin principle: short-term and long-term effects

Daniel says that adopting the diet changes suggested by the Pritikin Principle would certainly cause improvements in the short run for people switching from a standard American diet. But in the long run, extreme low-fat diets create many problems, not the least of which is the fact that most people can't stay on them. Those with enough willpower to stick with them are highly likely to develop health problems including low energy, inability to concentrate, depression, immune system breakdown, and even weight gain.

Like most diet plans, there are some good things to take from the Pritikin Principle, but there is no substitute for educating yourself about nutrition and making good choices that you can live with for a lifetime.

American nutritionist Nathan Pritikin came up with the idea of Pritikin diet in the 70's, mainly to combat his own cardiovascular ailment. This is why the diet mainly focuses on the consumption of unprocessed food groups, low in protein and fat, but rich in complex carbohydrates.

The Pritikin principle can be thought of as a super-low-fat-diet. While any healthy, balanced diet recommends putting fat at 20-30% of what you eat. The Pritikin weight loss program, on the other hand, keeps it under 10%. By keeping the fat consumption at an all-time low, the diet claims to help you lose weight while eating as much as you want.

The Pritikin principle is not only low in fat, it is loaded with complex carbohydrates as well. This diet encourages you to eat plenty if high-fiber grains, vegetables, and fruits frequently during the day. This approach helps you lose weight since you are curbing appetite by loading up on filling foods through the day and lowering your calorie intake. The Pritikin diet works best when you pair it with exercise and physical activity, as well as a strong social support and a stress-free life.

Unrefined complex carbohydrates

When on the Pritikin diet, it is recommended to consume 5 or more servings daily of:

• whole grains, such as millet, quinoa, barley, brown rice, rye, oats, and whole wheat

• starchy vegetables such as winter squashes, yams, and potatoes

• legumes, such as lentils, peas, and beans

Chestnuts

A serving means 1/2 cup cooked. As for whole-grain bread products such as crackers, bagels, and breads, one serving is 1 ounce. You must have noticed that the Pritikin diet doesn't encourage much white, but white doesn't always translate to unhealthy. For instance, non-fat yogurt, jicama, white potatoes, and cauliflower are all perfectly healthy foods.

Vegetables

The Pritikin diet recommends 5 servings of vegetables daily. A serving means ½ cup uncooked or 1 cup cooked. Mix in a wide variety of colors, like orange, red, yellow, green, purple. No need to count calories or your servings when you are consuming low-calorie-dense foods. You will shed off those extra pounds just by taking in less calories.

Fruits

You should take in at least four servings of fresh fruits daily on the Pritikin diet. A serving of fruit is anything that can fit in your hand. Try to eat a wide variety of fresh fruits, as well as canned fruits without added sugar. Don't let anyone tell you that fruit is fattening. People lose over 100 pounds over fruit-rich diets like Pritikin.

Dairy and Dairy Substitutes

2 servings of dairy foods daily. 1 serving constitutes a half cup of nonfat varieties of cottage cheese and ricotta cheese, 3/4 cup of nonfat yogurt or 1 cup of nonfat milk. Choose plain nonfat milk, not sugar-laden flavored varieties like chocolate. You can also opt for nonfat Lactaid. You can also consume dairy milk substitutes that resemble the nutritional goodness of nonfat cow's milk in terms of protein, B-12, Vitamins D, and calcium. Fortified soymilks are the best choice here. Rice and Almond milks are also preferable, since they are rich in B-12, calcium, and Vitamin D.

However, since they are a poor source of protein, so for every cup of rice or almond milk you drink, be sure to add a lean, protein-rich food such as 2 egg whites or a half cup of cooked legumes. Coconut milk is a big no, since it is a rich source of saturated fat. Make sure that all dairy milk substitutes are devoid of saturated fats, sodium, and sugars. On a side note, we have many plant-based calcium sources as well, such as tempeh, tofu, and green leafy vegetables such as kale, turnip greens, and collard greens.

Protein-Rich Foods

Being one of the healthiest diets you can follow, Pritikin advocates both animal and plant protein sources.

Protein-Rich Animal Foods:

• Consume no more than 1 serving (3½ to 4 ounces cooked) of Lean meat, Poultry, and Fish. Best protein sources include grass-fed and free-range elk, Venison, and bison, skinless white poultry, and omega-3-rich fish, such as Omega-3-rich fish, mackerel, sardines, and salmons at least twice daily.

• If you are a canned variety, choose a low sodium variety. Shelled mollusks, such as scallops, mussels, oysters and clams are also good, but don't eat much of crustaceans like lobster, crab, and shrimp.

• Steer clear of red meet, like goat, lamb, veal, pork, and beef, and select cuts that are under 30% fat.

• For optimal heart-health, don't eat red meat more than once a month.

Egg whites

Try to consume up to 2 egg whites a day. You can eat even more egg whites instead of land-based animal foods like meat and poultry. 1 serving of poultry or meat equals about 7 egg whites. However, try to avoid egg yolks since they are high in dietary cholesterol.

Protein-Rich Plant Foods

Legumes such as lentils, peas, beans, and soy products like edamame and tofu. If your goal is to reverse atherosclerosis or reduce your cholesterol levels, try to eat more of protein-rich plant foods instead of animal sources.

Beverages

While you are advised to get your recommended fill of water, you can enjoy herbal teas, such as chamomile, rosehips, peppermint, and green tea, coffee substitutes, and non-alkali processed hot cocoa. If you must have caffeinated beverages, we recommend that you drink black tea over coffee. Moderation is the key with this diet.

Drink up no more than 400 mg of caffeine daily, which comes down to 8 eight-ounce cups of tea or 4 eight-ounce cups of coffee. Be it decaf or regular, certain chemicals in coffee are known to raise the LDL cholesterol. However, you can mostly eliminate this chemical by brewing with paper filters.

Coffee, both regular and decaf, does contain chemicals (diterpenes) that may modestly raise LDL cholesterol. However, by brewing with paper filters like paper cones or capsule filters like Keurig, the diterpenes are largely eliminated.

Alcoholic beverages

Better to avoid all alcoholic beverages or consume in moderation. Up to 4 drinks are allowed in a day, but not more than 1 drink a day. A drink approximates 1½ oz of 80 proof liquor, 12 oz. of beer, or 5 oz. of wine. Red wine is the most suitable choice over other liquor types.

Herbs

Incorporate a wide array of herbs while on the Pritikin diet, since they are a rich source of phytonutrients, and add flavor to your food in place of salt and fat. Be sure to add at least 1 to 2 tablespoons of fresh herbs each day to your diet.

Artificial Sweeteners

Swap all sugar intake with artificial sweeteners. While they have no connection to weight loss, they are a great alternative for people on the Pritikin weight loss Plan, or even those with elevated triglycerides or diabetes. However, take no more than 10 to 12 packets per day. Two of the safest choices in this regard are stevia and sucralose.

What to avoid on the pritikin diet?

These foods fall in the "stop" category.Every time you are faced with one of these foods, run. All items belonging to this category are notorious for their high content of sodium, cholesterol, hydrogenated fat, and saturated fat, and can compromise your personal health goals. Sadly, most foods in an average American diet fit this description. Here's what to avoid while on the Pritikin Diet.

The typical american unhealthy diet

Steer far away from the typical American Diet, brimming over deep-fried foods, egg yolks, unhealthy oils, and fatty meats. Such an unhealthy diet is the root cause of heart ailments, high-cholesterol, obesity, hypertension, and type-. diabetes

Animal Fats, Processed Refined Oils and Tropical Oils

This includes margarine, chocolate, cocoa butter, chicken fat, lard, palm kernel oil, coconut oil, butter, shortenings, hydrogenated and partially hydrogenated vegetable oils.

Meats

• Such as processed meats, organ meats, and fatty meats.

• Whole and Low-Fat Dairy

• All cheese, sour cream, milk, ice cream, half and half, cream cheese, cream, and yogurt, unless fat-free and low in sodium.

• Nuts

• Salt Substitutes

• Miscellaneous

• Egg yolks, deep-fried foods, non-dairy whipped toppings, rich desserts and pastries, and salty snack foods.

Sample pritikin menu for 1 week

Day 1

• Breakfast: ½ cup whole-grain oats, cooked in low-fat milk, topped with sliced strawberries and bananas

• Midmorning Snack: 1 large tangerine, 1 steamed corn tortilla with fresh or grilled vegetables, one slice of fat free cheese, and salsa

• Lunch: Toss together 2 cups mixed greens with 1 cup of any other veggies, dressed with a dash of canola oil and aged balsamic vinegar. Serve with one ear of corn, and black Lentil soup.

• Midafternoon Snack: 1 apple

• Dinner: A bowl of fresh salad dressed with red wine vinegar, pan seared salmon with steamed broccoli and asparagus, and 1 baked potato with a dollop of fat-free sour cream,

Day 2

• Breakfast: Egg white omelet stuffed with broccoli, onions, spinach, and bell peppers, 1 bowl of fresh blueberries, and 1 cup cocoa.

• Midmorning Snack: grapes

• Lunch: Cream of crab and mushroom soup, A big bowl of salad tossed in with your favorite beans, and ½ whole-wheat bagel lightly buttered.

• Midafternoon Snack: 1 pear, 1 bowl of plain, non-fat yogurt

• Dinner: 1 cup cooked whole-wheat couscous, served with grilled herb roasted chicken, and a salad of fresh greens, avocado, and baby tomatoes.

Day 3

• Breakfast:

• Midmorning Snack: ½ cup whole-grain oats, cooked in low-fat milk, topped with blueberries, strawberries, and walnuts, 1 cup tea with non-fat milk and no sugar

• Midmorning Snack: 1 cup watermelon, 1 cucumber

• Lunch: Papaya salad, vegetable and bean soup, and Sandwich of whole-wheat bread, fresh roasted turkey breast and assorted veggies, dressed with nonfat mayonnaise and mustard.

• Midafternoon Snack: 2 cups air-popped popcorn or 1 cup fresh fruit salad

• Dinner: 1 veggie burger with whole wheat bun, served with roasted baby red potatoes, and romaine lettuce salad.

Day 4

• Breakfast: 1 cup low-fat yogurt mixed with 1 cup cubed fresh fruit, hash browns, with tea/coffee

• Midmorning Snack: Black bean salsa, with baked tortilla chips

• Lunch: A huge serving of salad incorporating mixed baby salad greens and assorted fresh veggies such as sliced jicama, tomatoes, avocados, and radishes, seasoned with red wine vinegar. A handful of strawberries. 1 serving of whole-wheat penne pasta with tomato and mushroom sauce.

• Midafternoon Snack: ½ cup fat-free cottage cheese mixed in with 1 cup fresh diced fruit

• Dinner: Black lentil soup, baby spinach salad dressed with balsamic red vinegar, tangy grilled chicken breast with grilled pine-apple slices and sweet potato chips.

Day 5

• Breakfast: ½ cup whole-grain oats, cooked in low-fat milk, topped with sliced blueberries and bananas

• Midmorning Snack: Celery sticks and carrot sticks with ½ cup red bean dip

• Lunch: Salad of mixed baby romaine lettuce seasoned with shrimp-cocktail-style dressing. 1 cup melon. Cream of crab and mushroom soup with baked potato.

• Midafternoon Snack: 1 pear, 1 bowl of plain, non-fat yogurt

• Dinner: 1 cup steamed kale seasoned with garlic and red pepper, served with sautéed garlic shrimp. 1 cup of white bean soup, and 3 cups of mixed baby salad greens tossed in with roasted red pepper and cucumber, dressed with canola oil and balsamic red wine vinegar.

Day 6

• Breakfast: Egg white omelet stuffed with mushrooms, onions, spinach, and bell peppers, 1 bowl of fresh blueberries, and 1 cup cocoa.

• Midmorning Snack: Corn tortilla, served with non-fat sour cream, corn kernels, and salsa. 1 apple.

• Lunch: Canned tuna or salmon, topped with crunchy spinach and non-fat mayo, served with crispbreads, 1 bowl raspberries, and 1 cup of carrot and cilantro soup.

• Midafternoon Snack: 1 bowl of grapes, and 1 bowl non-fat yogurt

• Dinner: 1 cup steamed asparagus, vegetable lasagna, a salad of mixed greens tossed in with cherry tomatoes and cannellini beans, dressed with canola oil and red wine vinegar.

Day 7

• Breakfast: ½ cup whole-grain oats, cooked in low-fat milk, topped with sliced blueberries and bananas, 1 glass orange juice

• Midmorning Snack: 6 whole-wheat low-sodium crackers with hummus dip

• Lunch: 1 grilled mushroom burger, 1 cup fresh fruits, and mixed salad greens

• Dinner: Cream of tomato soup, Greek-style salad with low-fat feta, and 1 cup cooked brown rice

Pritikin Diet

The Pritikin diet is a diet low in fats and high in complex carbohydrates.

What you can eat with the pritikin principle

The Pritikin Principle has more than 20 pages of charts listing the caloric density of many foods. The plan is to eat food that has a lot of fiber and water, such as vegetables, fruits, beans, and natural, unprocessed grains.

Pritikin doesn't have you counting calories, but you do have to know how to calculate the "average caloric density of your meal," and then keep that average below a certain number.

How the pritikin principle works

Pritikin suggests we eat whole, unprocessed, and natural carbohydrate-rich foods, such as grains, vegetables, and fruit. Preferred foods include:

• Brown rice

• Millet

• Barley

• Oats

• Dark green, leafy vegetables

• Onions

• Potatoes

• Squash

• Beans (black turtle beans, chickpeas, lentils, lima and pinto beans)

• Apples

• Pears

• Strawberries

• Bananas

• Some processed whole-grain foods, such as oatmeal, are OK on the plan. Even white-flour pasta is OK, as long as you eat it with vegetables.

Other guidelines:

• You can eat small portions of lean beef, chicken, and low-fat dairy products.

• Fish is fine, preferably three servings per week of salmon or other fish rich in omega-3 fatty acids.

• Avoid fried foods, dressing with fat, and fatty sauces.

• Eat three meals a day plus two snacks.

• Stay active and avoid salty foods.

• Artificial sweeteners are OK on the plan, too

Recipe

Creamy Chicken Ravoli Soup

Introduction

• Creamy chicken soup with ravoli-Easy soup half the time by using rotesserie chicken

• Minutes to Prepare: 20

• Minutes to Cook: 60

• Number of Servings: 11

Ingredients

• 2 tbsp olive oil

• 1/4 chopped onion

• 1/4 chopped celery

• 1/4 chopped carrots

• 1.5 cup chopped rotesserie chicken

- 1 can of fat free cream of chicken soup

- 2 32 oz container of chicken broth

- 1 jar of ragu alfredo sauce

- 1// bag of round cheese ravoli

Directions

- This will make about 11 cups of soup

- Saute your onion, carrot, and celery until soft and clear

- Add chicken to sauteed veggies

- add chicken broth

- add cream of chick soup

- add alfredo

- add cheese ravoli

- Stir together and bring to a boil

- Redcue heat and simmer for an 1 hr to 45 minutes

Homemade Chicken Salad

Introduction

• homade chicken salad made from leftover fried chicken

• Minutes to Prepare: 15

• Number of Servings: 8

Ingredients

• chicken removed from bone

• celery

• onion

• light mircle whip

• bread

• Directions

• Remove chicken from the bone. Add celery, onion, and mircle whip. Mix all together. spread onto bread.

Spicy Southern Barbecued Chicken

Introduction

• Removing the chicken fat and skin and adding no salt to the tasty sauce makes this chicken favorite heart-healthy.

Ingredients

- 3 lb. chicken parts (breast, drumstick, and thigh), skin and fat removed

- 1 large onion, thinly sliced

- 3 tablespoon vinegar

- 3 tablespoon Worcestershire sauce

- 2 tablespoon brown sugar

- black pepper to taste

- 1 tablespoon hot pepper flakes

- 1 tablespoon chili powder

- 1 cup chicken stock or broth, skim fat from top

Directions

1. Place chicken in a 13x9x2" pan. Arrange onions over the top.

2. Mix together vinegar, Worcestershire sauce, brown sugar, pepper, hot pepper flakes, chili powder, and stock.

3. Pour over the chicken and bake at 350º F for 1 hour or until done.

4. Baste occasionally.

Yield: 8 servings--Serving Size: One chicken part with sauce

Tastey Cream of Chicken Chicken Tenderloins

Introduction

• This can give you all the taste of baked chicken and rice but lets you cook the chicken on the skillet instead of baking.

• Minutes to Prepare: 5

• Minutes to Cook: 25

• Number of Servings: 1

Ingredients

• 2 Chicken Tenderloins or Breast cut up

• 1 Can Campbells Low Fat Cream of Chicken Soup

• Directions

• Cook chicken until brown.You will want to cut up the chicken tenderloins or breasts into smaller pieces for faster cook time. Add the cream of chicken soup and simmer for about 10 minutes.

• Top this on a bed of brown rice and enjoy!

Potato Flake Fried Chicken (Breast)

Introduction

• Adjusted recipe entered by SPICEAHOLIC for 1 pound of chicken breast instead of 1.5 pounds of chicken thigh.

• Minutes to Prepare: 10

• Minutes to Cook: 25

• Number of Servings: 4

Ingredients

• 16 oz Chicken Breast, boneless skinless

• 1 c Instant Mashed Potato Flakes

• Butter Substitute, Spray

Directions

• Pre-heat oven to 350 degrees Farenheit.

• Line baking sheet with foil and spray with cooking spray.

• Place potato flakes in large bowl. Add whatever seasonings you'd like.

• Spray each side of chicken breast with spray , then coat with potato flakes. Make sure to coat thoroughly.

• Place flaked bresats on baking sheet. Sprinkle remaining flakes as desired over chicken. Spray tops with cooking spray.

• Bake for about 25 minutes or until cooked through.

• Makes 4 servings (4 oz chicken breast each)

Beverages

• You'll drink mainly water, herbal tea or coffee substitutes on the Pritikin diet, though you can also have 1 cup of caffeinated coffee or 3 cups of caffeinated tea each day.

• Women can have up to four alcoholic beverages weekly, while men can have up to seven.

Black Bean Sauce For Ravioli

Ingredients

• 2 cups dry black beans

• 8 cups vegetable stock (low-sodium)

• onion chopped

• red bell pepper chopped

• green bell pepper chopped

• leeks white only chopped

• 1/2 cup ketchup (unsweetened)

• tablespoons garlic chopped

• 1 teaspoon soy sauce, low sodium

• teaspoon tofu parmesan

• 1/4 teaspoon cumin

• 1/4 teaspoon coriander

• 1/4 teaspoon black pepper

• 1/4 teaspoon crushed red pepper

Instructions

• Soak the beans in water for 8 hours or overnight, placing the pan in the refrigerator so that the beans will not ferment.

• Before cooking the beans, drain the soaking liquid and rinse the beans with clean water.

• Put the beans on the stovetop in a large pot, such as a Dutch oven.

• Add the vegetable stock, onion, bell peppers, and leeks.

• Bring the beans and veggies to a boil and then reduce to a simmer, partially covering the pot.

• If any foam develops, you can skim it off during the simmering process. Black beans generally take about 1½ to 2 hours to become very soft.

When very soft, puree.

• Add remaining ingredients, stir, and serve.

Creamed Spinach

Ingredients

• 1 medium onion finely chopped

• 1 teaspoon garlic finely chopped

• 1 pound spinach (frozen) thawed, and drained

- 1/2 teaspoon Pritikin All-Purpose Seasoning (homemade blend of granulated onion, granulated garlic, salt-free lemon pepper, and paprika)

- 1 dash nutmeg ground

- 2 tablespoons white wine optional

- 1.5 cups milk nonfat

- 2 tablespoons veggie topping

- 1 tablespoon cornstarch dissolved in 2 tablespoons cold water

- 2 tablespoons sour cream, fat free or fat-free plain yogurt

- 1 medium tomato diced

- 1 optional artichoke when available

Instructions

- Sauté onion and garlic until translucent. Season spinach with all-purpose seasoning and nutmeg.

- Add spinach to onion and garlic. Sauté and cook for 3 minutes. Add white wine (optional), nonfat milk, and 1 tablespoon veggie topping. Cook for another 4 minutes.

• Thicken spinach mixture with cornstarch. Then add sour cream. Lower flame and stir constantly until mixture is creamy.

• Add remaining veggie topping and serve, garnished with diced tomatoes and artichoke stems, if available.

Tortilla Dessert Cups

Ingredients

• For the tortilla cups:

• 3 10-inch flour tortillas

• 2 tablespoons butter, melted

• ¼ cup sugar

• 1 tablespoon cinnamon

• For the whipped cream:

• 1 cup heavy whipping cream

• 2 tablespoons sugar

• 1 teaspoon vanilla extract

• For topping:

• Fresh fruit

Preparation

1. Preheat oven to 375°F/190°C.

2. Butter each side of the tortillas, sprinkle with cinnamon sugar, and cut into even quarters, making 12 pieces.

3. Place two pieces in each cup of a muffin tin and push down so that it creates a cup shape.

4. Bake for 13-15 minutes or until crisp.

5. In a bowl, mix together heavy cream, vanilla extract, and sugar.

6. Assemble the cups by placing a spoonful of whipped cream in the toasted cup.

7. Top with fresh fruits of your choice.

8. Enjoy!

15 Minute Healthy Roasted Chicken and Veggies (One Pan)

Ingredients

- 2 medium chicken breasts chopped

- 1 cup bell pepper chopped (any colors you like)

- 1/2 onion chopped

- 1 zucchini chopped

- 1 cup broccoli florets

- 1/2 cup tomatoes chopped or plum/grape

- 2 tablespoons olive oil

- 1/2 teaspoon salt

- 1/2 teaspoon black pepper

- 1 teaspoon italian seasoning

- 1/4 teaspoon optional

Instructions

- Preheat oven to 500 degree F.

- Chop all the veggies into large pieces. In another cutting board chop the chicken into cubes. Place the chicken and veggies in a medium roasting dish or sheet pan. Add the olive oil, salt and pepper, italian seasoning, and paprika. Toss to combine.

• Bake for 15 minutes or until the veggies are charred and chicken is cooked. Enjoy with rice, pasta, or a salad

Mushroom, spring onion and baby broccoli stir-fry

• Marinade

• 1/4 cup olive oil

• 1 tbsp fresh thyme, finely chopped

• 2 shallots, finely chopped

• 1/2 cup oyster sauce

• 1/2 cup rice wine vinegar

• 500g portabella mushrooms, gills removed with a spoon Stir-fry

• 200g baby broccoli, ends trimmed

• 1 tbsp olive oil 4 spring onions, cut into 4cm pieces

• 1 tbsp finely chopped ginger

• 2 cloves garlic, finely chopped

• 2 tsp sesame seeds

Directions

• Preheat oven to 200C (180C fan forced).

• Mix all marinade ingredients except mushrooms in a large bowl.

• Add the mushrooms and coat well with the marinade.

• Place mushrooms stem-side down on a lined baking tray.

• Roast for 30 mins or until tender.

• Set aside to cool. Cut into 1cm slices.

• Refresh in iced water Drain.

• Place a large frying pan or wok over high heat and add the oil.

• When oil is very hot, add baby broccoli and cook for 2 mins or until bright green and beginning to char in spots.

• Add the mushrooms and toss to incorporate.

• Add spring onions, ginger and garlic and cook for 3-4 mins or until beans are tender.

• Add half the sesame seeds and season with salt and pepper.

• Serve on large platter and garnish with remaining sesame seeds.

Spinach and Kale Salad with Honey Dijon Vinaigrette

Ingredients

• About 8 cups baby spinach and baby kale combined

• 4 hard boiled eggs peeled and chopped

• 1 avocado cubed

• 4 small ripe tomatoes, quartered

• 1/4 medium red onion sliced

• 4 ounces feta cheese crumbled

• 4 tablespoons roasted sunflower seeds

• 4 tablespoons hulled hemp seeds

• 2 tablespoons Dijon mustard

• 2 tablespoons honey

• 1/4 cup apple cider vinegar

• 1 clove garlic minced

- 1/2 teaspoon fine sea salt

- 1/4 teaspoon ground black pepper

- 1/2 cup extra virgin olive oil

Instructions

- Either on a large serving platter or divided onto four dinner plates, arrange the spinach and kale and top with the remaining ingredients, up to the hemp seeds.

- In a small bowl or in a jar with a tight fitting lid, combine the dressing ingredients and either whisk or shake until emulsified.

- Top the salad with the dressing just before serving. Store any additional dressing covered in the fridge.

Bison with Mushrooms and Onions Recipe

Cooking Tips

- For grass-fed bison tenderloin cuts, chef Anthony7 says, "The cooking time should be short and fast.

- Because the meat does not have any marble (fat pockets), searing at high temps on each side for 90 seconds creates a nice crust and seals the juices Let the meat sit for another 2 to 3 minutes, and it will cook more, reaching a medium rare doneness.

• For grass-fed meat products, we do not recommend cooking beyond medium doneness because they will become rubbery due to the lack of fat."

• 4 four-ounce grass-fed, free-range bison steaks

• ½ pound button mushrooms, cleaned and sliced

• ½ pound shiitake mushrooms, cleaned and sliced

• 4 garlic cloves, finely sliced

• ½ pound onions, thinly sliced

• 1 ounce balsamic vinegar

• ¼ cup red wine

• ¼ cup Knudsen® Low-Sodium Very Veggie Juice

• 1 teaspoon chopped fresh thyme leaves

• 1 teaspoon chopped fresh tarragon

• Heat a large nonstick sauté pan over high heat. Sear bison for about 90 seconds per side, or until a crust is formed, but the meat is not fully cooked. Remove bison from pan and set aside.

• Add mushrooms, garlic, and onions to the pan; sauté until soft and lightly browned, about 4 minutes.

• Deglaze pan with vinegar. (To deglaze: Pour vinegar into pan, then gently scrape bottom of pan with a wooden spoon to loosen the caramelized juices.)

• Add wine, Knudsen® Low-Sodium Very Veggie Juice, thyme, and tarragon. Simmer for two minutes.

• Add bison steaks back to pan and simmer until bison is cooked through.

Butternut Squash Maple Walnut Scones

Dry Ingredients

• 11⁄2 cups (198 g) whole wheat pastry our (use a gluten-free baking mix)

• 3/4 cup (72 g) rolled oats

• 1⁄4 cup (60 g) coconut sugar or brown sugar

- 1 tablespoon (15 g) baking powder

- 1 teaspoon cinnamon

- 1/4 teaspoon nutmeg

- 1/2 teaspoon salt

Wet Ingredients

- 1/2 cup (123 g) butternut squash purée (you can use canned pumpkin in place of the butternut squash)

- 2 tablespoons (14 g) ground flax-seed mixed with 4 tablespoons (60 ml) warm water

- 1/4 cup (60 ml) nondairy milk

- 1/4 cup (60 ml) maple syrup

- 1 teaspoon maple extract

- 1/2 cup (55 g) chopped walnuts

Directions

- Preheat the oven to 350°F (176°C) and oil a large cookie sheet (or line with parchment).

• Mix the dry ingredients in a large mixing bowl. Mix the wet ingredients in a smaller bowl.

• Right before baking, add the wet ingredients into the dry ones and mix until thoroughly combined, then mix in the walnuts.

• Scoop out the batter to the middle of your prepared cookie sheet and pat it into a big circle about 3/4-inch thick. Using a chef 's knife, score into 12 triangles by cutting halfway through the dough.

• Bake for 25 to 30 minutes until golden brown.

Pumpkin Scone

• 2 cups of flour, plus more for dusting

• 1/3 cup lightly packed light brown sugar

• 1 tsp baking powder

• ¾ tsp ground cinnamon

• ½ tsp baking soda

• ½ tsp ground ginger

• ¼ tsp sea salt

- ½ cup cold unsalted butter, cut into pieces

- ½ cup cold buttermilk

- ½ cup pumpkin pureé

- ½ cup dried cranberries soaked in hot water for about 15 – 30 minutes and then drained, plumps and softens them up

- ½ tsp pure vanilla extract

- candied ginger finely chopped

- ¼ cup heavy cream

Directions

- Preheat the oven to 375 degrees and line a baking sheet with parchment paper.

- Whisk together the flour, sugar, baking powder, cinnamon, baking soda, ginger and salt in a large bowl. Cut the butter into the mixture until it resembles coarse meal.

- Whisk together the buttermilk, pumpkin and vanilla in a medium bowl until smooth. Add the wet mixture to the dry along with the cranberries and candied ginger. Mix until it is all just combined (do not over-mix or the scones will be tough).

• Transfer to a lightly-floured surface and knead the dough gently 4 or 5 times. Pat the dough into a circle that is about 8 inches round and about 1 1/2 inches thick. Cut the circle in half, and then cut each half into 4 pie-shaped wedges (triangles). Place the scones on the baking sheet and brush the tops with the heavy cream.

• Bake until golden brown and a toothpick inserted in the middle comes out with a few moist crumbs attached, 20 to 25 minutes. Let cool on a baking rack for 15 minutes before serving.

• Serve plain or goes great with maple butter or powder sugar drizzle icing and with a cup of tea.

Rocket Donuts' Blueberry Fritter

• Yeast Raised Dough

• 2 cups milk

• ½ oz dry active yeast

• 1 cup + 2 Tbs. sugar

• 8 cup all purpose flour

• 6 Tbs. butter

Directions

• Heat milk in a sauce pan and bring to a simmer. Pour into a mixing bowl to cool. In a separate bowl, pour yeast into a small amount of warm (not hot) water and let rest for 5 minutes. Pour yeast mixture into milk. Stir in 2 T of sugar. Add 3 cups all purpose flour to mixture and mix all ingredients for about 1-2 minutes. Cover bowl with a wet towel and let rise for 1 hour.

• After an hour, soften 6 T of butter. Mix ½ cup sugar with the butter. Add the butter sugar mixture to the covered mixture.

• Add 5 cups of flour and mix for 20-30 minutes on low speed. Pan and cover for an hour.

Blueberry Compote

• 1 lb blueberries

• 1 ¾ cups sugar

• 5 Tbs. corn starch

• Mash blueberries in a bowl. Place mashed blueberries into a heavy bottomed pot on low-to-medium heat. Add sugar until dissolved. Bring to a light boil. Add cornstarch until thick (stir for 2 minutes). Take off heat.

Glaze

- 4 oz hot water

- 3 ½ cups powdered Sugar

Fritters

- 4 lbs yeast raised dough

- 1 ½ cup blueberries

- ¾ cup blueberry compote

- ¼ cup flour

- Deep fryer oil (i.e. vegetable oil, shortening, peanut oil, coconut oil). Use enough oil to submerge fritters.

Directions

- Flatten dough and evenly spread compote on top. Sprinkle 1 ½ cups blueberries over blueberry compote and sift and fold 1/4 cup flour into dough.

- After folding all of the ingredients in, chop dough mixture thoroughly. Form chopped ingredients back into a ball and chop again (repeat this step 4 times).

• Use an ice cream scoop to portion into balls. Slightly flatten dough onto fryer screen by using fingers (tops should be bumpy). Proof the dough for 45 minutes.

• Preheat oil to 350 degrees. Submerge fritters in oil for 4 ½ minutes. Glaze while hot. Serve and enjoy!!

Creamy Chicken Ravoli Soup

Introduction

• Creamy chicken soup with ravoli-Easy soup half the time by using rotesserie chicken

• Minutes to Prepare: 20

• Minutes to Cook: 60

• Number of Servings: 11

Ingredients

• 2 tbsp olive oil

• 1/4 chopped onion

• 1/4 chopped celery

• 1/4 chopped carrots

- 1.5 cup chopped rotesserie chicken

- 1 can of fat free cream of chicken soup

- 2 32 oz container of chicken broth

- 1 jar of ragu alfredo sauce

- 1// bag of round cheese ravoli

Directions

- This will make about 11 cups of soup

- Saute your onion, carrot, and celery until soft and clear

- Add chicken to sauteed veggies

- add chicken broth

- add cream of chick soup

- add alfredo

- add cheese ravoli

- Stir together and bring to a boil

- Redcue heat and simmer for an 1 hr to 45 minutes

Grilled Beer Can Chicken

Ingredients

- 1 whole fryer chicken 4-5 #

- 1/2 can Budweiser beer

- 2-4 tsp of Grillmates Chicken rub

Directions

- clean chicken, rinse under cold water. remove bag inside chicken cavity.

- use 1/2 can of budweiser per chicken

- sprinkle chicken with grillmates chicken rub inside and out

- put chicken ontop of can and put a potatoe in the neck

- put chicken on grill

- grill 2-3 hours.

Oven Fried Chicken

Ingredients

- 6 skinless chicken legs (any part of chicken you choose)

- 1/2 cup skim milk

- 1/2 dry bread crumbs

- 1/3 cup grated parmesan cheese salt and pepper dash (to taste)

Directions

Heat oven to 375 degrees remove skin from chicken,place chicken in a shallow pan. Pour milk over chicken and then refrigerate while you prepare the coating mix. In shallow bowl mix breadcrumbs,cheese,salt,and pepper.Roll chicken around in breadcrumb mix,coating chicken well. Place chicken on a slightly greased baking sheet place in oven bake at 375 degrees for 45 minutes.

Chicken Quesidilla

Ingredients

- 1 chicken thigh-boneless and skinless

- 1 96% fat free flour tortilla

- 1/4 2% colby & monterey jack shredded cheese

- 1 tbsp litgh sour cream

Directions

• Heat 1 tbsp olive oil in pan to cook chicken. Be sure to cook chicken thoroghly. Season chicken with a little garlic powder, onion powder, season salt, and pepper. Cook chicken until brown on both sides.

• Melt cheese on tortilla.

• Cut cooked chicken into strips and place on tortilla

• Add sour cream and/or salsa on top of chicken. Roll up and enjoy.

Indonesian Peanut Chicken

Ingredients

• 1 large, whole chicken breat, cut into bite-sized pieces

• salt & pepper

• 1 tbsp. canola or vegetable oil

• 1 med. yellow onion, finely diced

• 1/4 cup peanut butter (preferrably organic)

• 1/3 cup chili sauce

- 1 cup water

- 1 med. red bell pepper chopped

- handful of peanuts

- 2 cups of rice- cooked

Directions

- Makes 4-6 servings

- Sprinkle Chicken with salt and pepper, heat oil over med-high heat in a large pan

- Saute chicken until lightly browned on all sides and just opaquue throughout

- Place chicken on a plate, saute onion until softened in chicken drippings

- Once onion is soft add peanut butter and chili sauce to pan, reduce heat to medium

- gradually stir in water until peanut butter is melted and sauce is fully blended

- add chicken back to pan until mixture heats through

• Serve chicken and sauce mixture over rice, topped with bell pepper and peanuts

Grilled Chipotle Chicken Breasts

Ingredients

• 5 chipotle peppers, seeded and chopped by hand

• 1-3 cup cilantro leaves

• 2 cloves garlic

• 2 medium shallots

• 1/3 cup rice vinegar

• 1/4 cup olive oil

• Juice of 2 limes

• 2 chicken breasts

Directions

1. Purée the peppers, cilantro, garlic, shallots and vinegar in a food processor or blender. With the machine running add the oil slowly and then the lime juice. This will be the marinade for your chicken.

2. Divide the marinade into two portions- one to marinate your chicken and another (in a separate container or bowl) to baste your chicken later while it cooks.

3. Marinate the chicken for approximately 1 to 3 hours or overnight. Remove chicken from marinade and grill slowly over medium fire. Discard marinade used by the chicken (for food safety) and baste the chicken with excess marinade that was set aside.

Lemon Chicken

Ingredients

- 4 boneless, skinless chicken breasts

- 2 teaspoons dried basil leaves

- 2 tablespoons chopped fresh parsley

- 2 tablespoons lemon juice

- 2 teaspoons olive oil

- 1/2 teaspoon salt

- 1 garlic clove, finely chopped

Directions

1. Remove fat from chicken.

2. Make lemon sauce: Beat remaining ingredients in a medium-sized bowl with a whisk or fork.

3. Spray a 10-inch skillet with cooking spray and cook chicken over medium-high heat for about 15 minutes or until juices are no longer pink when thickest part of chicken is cut.

4. Spoon some lemon sauce over chicken, turn chicken over and cook for an additional 15-20 seconds. Serve chicken topped with remainder of sauce.

www.ingramcontent.com/pod-product-compliance
Lightning Source LLC
Chambersburg PA
CBHW051359150726
48000CB00003B/1251